A heartfelt thanks to my twin sister, Penny Nelson for her contribution to the material and her lifetime of support and encouragement; to Kathleen Elmore, my friend and mentor, for the gift of grace through her spiritual guidance, her belief in me, and her editing skills; to Barbara Cady who through her years of friendship and association as a business partner taught me a kinder, gentler approach; to Meredith Young-Sowers for her teachings of the human energy system which opened up in me the creative foundation for this work; to Carol Allen for her friendship, her ability to keep me on track, and contribution to the technical aspects; and to my friend Judy Henry for her time and expertise in adapting and formatting the illustrations.

To Pat
I love you!
Pam
12/25/2012

Table of Contents

Introduction – My Story

The Art of Heart Healing sprang from the knowledge, wisdom and experience of my 30 plus years as a coronary care nurse combined with my study of the human energy system. The result is a profound understanding of the relationship of the physical and emotional heart.

I have been a student of the heart my entire life. I now understand that I began my study of the emotional heart as a young child. My father was an alcoholic, and my mom was a product of the 1930's and 40's when culture dictated that families stay together no matter what. I know my coping mechanisms would have been fewer had it not been for my identical twin sister, Penny, with whom I have shared the emotions of my life as they have unfolded. I now know the plan was to experience and observe many angles of emotions of the heart, and my higher education continued with a devastating divorce in my 20's from my high school sweetheart, and the death of my longtime partner eleven years ago. He died predictably of heart disease.

I began my formal education in this field at age seventeen as a nursing student. Because my interest has always been in cardiology, I began working in coronary care units from their inception in the 60's. I continued to learn about heart disease and the emotions that accompany this disease throughout the next thirty-three years as a coronary nurse in various hospitals including Baylor and Stanford.

My interest in the human energy system began when Penny and I decided to take a Healing Touch™ class about fifteen years ago. She too was a coronary nurse, and we decided we were bored with continuing education courses about cardiology. This workshop was an introduction to an approach to wellness we had not considered. In CCU we saw patients return time after time with the same symptoms. Much is known about how to treat acute conditions and save lives in the short term, but patients with the diagnosis of heart disease often suffer reoccurrences because the underlying problems remain. All those years as a nurse when asked "How do I prevent another heart attack?" I would love to have had a definitive answer. To understand and explain that emotion can play a part in decreased energy flow of the heart and restoring that flow can play a huge role in restoring heart health, would have given people options and hope.

I've been inspired by many patients over the years, but one patient really stands out. I cared for this patient as a cardiac nurse over about a ten year period. His name was Pat. He began having heart attacks in his 20's. He had a family history of heart attacks, and his family and siblings died at a young age. He was married and had three daughters. Over that ten year period, the entire staff got to know him and his family really well. We shared holidays, birthday parties, anniversaries and even a prom, because he was in the hospital so frequently with chest pain. Over the course of the years he had two bypass surgeries and numerous angioplasties with stints. He received clot busting medication to dissolve clots in coronary arteries; averting heart attacks so many times I lost count. He went to specialists all over the country always searching for the answer. He couldn't work. He couldn't do any activity that exerted his heart, or he would have chest pain. He finally opted for experimental surgery. It was done in the Medical Center of Houston. We learned he arrested during the surgery, and although the doctors were able to revive him, he died two days later. Through my sadness, I began to ask what was missing. I've come to know that we failed to address the emotions of his heart.

The doctors and nurses were desperate to help this man. Science went as far as it could. *The Art of Heart Healing* furnishes the missing link to creating wellness. The combination of state of the art medical care, learning about the underlying emotions of heart disease, and energetically rewiring your subconscious through awareness of how it works is an awesome combination with unlimited potential.

In my enthusiasm to learn more about the energy system of the body and the effect of emotions on the physical body, I have studied Healing Touch for people and animals and also, such disciplines as Reiki, Melchizedek Method, Integrated Energy Techniques, Angelic Healing, Huna, Matrix Energetics, The Reconnection, The One Command and have attended the Angel Guide School of Light. In 2001, I graduated from The Stillpoint School of Advanced Energy Healing as a Certified Intuitive Healer.

The school of thought in the medical field is if you have a history of heart disease you'll just have to live with the genetics you've been dealt. There is nothing you can do about it. However, that is changing. I've learned people come to this life with other souls who agree to work on common issues. In science that's called heredity.

Kathleen Elmore, my friend and mentor, has been a great inspiration and a catalyst for much I have learned. She has taught me that many people of our generation have said, "the buck stops here". Kathleen is the founder of *The Angel Guide School of Light,* of which I am a graduate. More information about her can be found at www.angelways.com.

Her teachings inspired what I call Generational Healing. This is healing that makes possible life-changes on a level that not only impacts you but generations past and future. We live in exciting times. The energy of the planet has changed, and we have evolved so these changes are accessible. When healing takes place at this level, DNA is impacted.

Thank you for joining me on this journey of sharing what I've learned in my 30 plus years of studying the incredible workings and wisdom of the heart.

Basis for Art of Heart Healing

Welcome to *The Art of Heart Healing*! Heart problems are an invitation to make changes in your life so that you can live a meaningful life in which love and peace fill and surround you. Imbalances manifested by heart disease are opportunities to examine how you are living. Your particular difficulties illuminate the areas of focus which you are subconsciously longing to bring into balance. Doing this will enhance your spiritual, emotional, and physical well being. By following your doctor's orders AND working the program outlined here, you will find yourself living a more meaningful, satisfying life than ever before.

I'll tell you a little about how *The Art of Heart Healing* came about. As I expressed before, it has been my experience and frustration as a nurse that there is no cure for heart disease. I began to realize that people kept coming back with the same symptoms related to the heart because we literally never got to the heart of the problem. In my pursuit to understand the dynamics of why people didn't heal long term, I decided to learn more about the energy system of the body. I studied with Meredith Young-Sowers at *The Stillpoint School of Advanced Energy Training* for nine months. Her amazing work around the energy centers of the body and how they relate to our beliefs and subsequent emotions around events in our lives was invaluable. What I've come to know is: The heart is **Command Central** of the body.

Let's start with some background information. Science supports the fact that we are energy beings. Traditional science recognizes we are made of energy and has documented that our bodies are made up of molecules that are constantly in motion. Quantum physics came into being in the 1920's, and energy has gradually come to the forefront as the focus of the composition of our world and everything in it. Before Quantum physics, we constructed our thinking according to Newtonian physics which concentrated more on matter. This led to taking things apart in order to repair them rather than considering the whole. That continues to be the basis of most traditional medicine today although there is some progress toward holism. An example is stem cell therapy. Stem cells take on the characteristics of the environment in which they are placed. This is an example of how everything is interconnected. No longer can we treat only a part without considering the whole because energy is boundless.

From an energy standpoint, our bodies, as well as all living things, are surrounded by an electromagnetic field that has vibrational frequency. The human energy field looks like an inverted egg and can extend out several feet from the physical body. You may have been aware of your own energy field when someone else was "in your space." That's exactly what happened. Another person was literally standing in your energy field, and their energy field was interacting with yours.

The heart itself is also surrounded by an electromagnetic field. This field has been researched extensively by the Institute of HeartMath®. The HeartMath Institute is an organization that has done much research to scientifically prove what has been intuitively suspected for eons. They have shown that the heart is the biggest generator of electromagnetic energy in the body - even more than the brain. Because it is the biggest generator of electromagnetic energy and is the largest oscillating organ in the body, the other organs can synchronize with the heart.[i] That is why the state of your heart is important to the state of the rest of your body.

Your system is the microcosm of the macrocosm of the Universe. Your heart is the center of your Universe, and everything rotates around it, just as in our solar system. I recently went to a production of *The Planets* at the Houston Symphony. Gustav Holst composed this music in England between 1914 and 1916. The symphony accompanied this music composed in the early part of the last century with contemporary pictures of the solar system taken by the Hubble telescope and Voyager. The pictures were shown on a big screen while the symphony played the music, and the results were dramatic and moving. It really brought home to me the divine order of things. That same divine order lives in our bodies and is dependent upon the integrity of our individual solar system whose center around which everything else revolves and evolves. The center of our personal Universe is the heart.

Every function of the body revolves around the function of the heart. I learned working as a nurse that when the heart began to fail, every other system of the body began to fail. When the energy of the heart is altered or muted and does not flow smoothly, the heart will function poorly. Eventually its poor performance affects the performance of all other organs.

You may wonder what would keep energy from flowing smoothly through your energy system. Energy is constantly moving and has a vibrational frequency like a wave of light or a sound wave. Just as a light source can be blocked by an object, the flow of energy can be blocked by alterations in the configuration of the energy field. Alterations can be caused by the pollution of our energy field. This pollution may be a result of things we consume such as food, alcohol, drugs, air or unreleased emotions such as anger or grief.

In the world of energy, everything starts out as finer matter (thoughts and feelings) and then if it persists, becomes denser energy and can manifest in the physical. That's why it's really important to monitor your thoughts. Today's thoughts are tomorrow's reality. So it makes good sense to look at the energetic picture that underlies the overt forms of disease. Without exploring the emotional cause of illness, we may be pruning the diseased branches with our band aid approach to medicine, but not healing the root of the problem. This may sustain life, but fail when it comes to achieving quality of life.

Another factor that can alter our energy field is stress. Health care providers have known for some time that stress itself is a major cause of illness and that lowering levels of stress is vital to our health. Yet how to accomplish this can often be a stress itself. This program will teach you how to identify those feelings that are not in alignment with your heart's inherent peaceful energy. This focus will bring your entire body into the energy of peace.

The purpose of this handbook is to pass on what I've learned about *The Art of Heart Healing.* It is an approach that combines my experiences and education as a nurse with my study of energy to define the relationship of the physical heart to the emotional heart. This is the key to discerning the emotional causes of heart disease. My desire in sharing this information is to offer hope in the regeneration of the heart when often there is little. The following is an overview of how the heart works and how that relates to energy.

The upper chambers of the heart are the atria. They are the "receiving" chambers -- one receives blood from the body and the other receives oxygenated or nourished blood from the lungs. The ventricles are the lower chambers and are the "giving" chambers of the heart. One gives blood to the lungs to be oxygenated; the other gives oxygenated or nourished blood to itself and the body. This combined with what I learned from Meredith Young-Sowers at Stillpoint, that the right side of the heart has to do with self love and the left side with love for others (partner, family, friend) is the fundamental basis for *The Art of Heart Healing*. These principals will be more fully developed as I discuss each condition and disease individually.

This program is designed to allow you to take the symptoms of a condition, build them together like components of a sound system to individualize the understanding of what's energetically underlying the disease, and thus tailor the treatment program to meet your individual needs. You will see that in using *The*

Art of Heart-Healing Handbook, the more information you have about what part of your heart is affected, the more definitive your understanding will be as to where to look in your life for answers. If you have coronary artery disease, it is important to get as much information as possible about the involved part of the heart. Ask for copies of test results. Even if you don't understand the medical lingo, the summary will allow you to look it up, or ask someone for further explanation. I really encourage you to be proactive in your treatment. As a practicing nurse, I found that if patients had an understanding of what was involved, they could often make very good intuitive decisions about what approach was right for them.

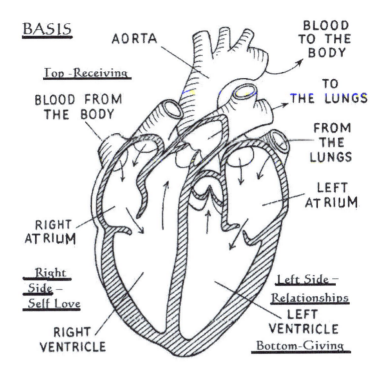

BASIS

AORTA

BLOOD TO THE BODY

Top - Receiving

BLOOD FROM THE BODY

TO THE LUNGS

FROM THE LUNGS

LEFT ATRIUM

RIGHT ATRIUM

Right Side – Self Love

Left Side – Relationships

LEFT VENTRICLE

RIGHT VENTRICLE

Bottom-Giving

Heart Attacks and Angina

From an energy standpoint, heart attacks and angina occur when nourishment to the heart muscle becomes diminished because of narrowing of the coronary arteries due to blockage or spasm. The coronary arteries supply the heart muscle with oxygenated blood. The decreased nourishment or blood supply may cause weakness or even death of the heart muscle. When this occurs, the weakened heart muscle is unable to be exercised for its intended purpose which is circulating vitality to itself and the body. From a broader perspective this translates to less vibrancy due to a narrowed connection not only to oneself but to the whole. Starving heart muscle or decreased blood flow is manifested by pain also known as angina which I will address first as it can be a precursor to a heart attack. Death of the heart muscle occurs when the blood supply, or nourishment, is cut off completely, and that is what is commonly called a heart attack.

Angina - a precursor to heart attacks

Angina is pain generated by insufficient oxygen supplied to the heart muscle because of diminished flow. Flow is important – both what flows in and what flows out. This is a reflection of how you manage your everyday life. Are you able to be in the flow and adjust to changes as they occur, or are you always pushing, insisting it must work the way it always has or how you think it should? This decreased flow can be a result of narrowed arteries or spasms (uncertainty) in the arteries. Energetically, a narrowed flow represents a narrowed view. We see only our human self in a small sense rather than our eternal soul in a bigger picture. This does not allow the flow of all that we are to fulfill our heart's desire -- which is to freely share our gifts with the world. The resulting effect is the pain of feeling that we are not fulfilling our mission or purpose in life, and we may blame either ourselves or others. Angina calls for the need to look at self empowerment and self acceptance. Self acceptance opens the door to accepting others. Angina is heart pain that represents a starving heart. Communication with your heart is cut off because of a narrowed view of oneself as merely a physical body going through the motions of a physical life rather than a spiritual being fulfilling one's spiritual contract (heart's desire)

Heart Attack (Myocardial Infarction)

Myocardial infarction (MI) is the medical term for heart attack. I am always amazed at how the terms of medical conditions often intuitively allude to the energy of the condition. A heart "attack" -- who could attack our hearts but ourselves? We are fond of blaming others for our feelings, but it's an inside job.

Anterior MI

An anterior MI (myocardial infarction) is damage to the anterior or front wall of the heart. This heart attack involves the Left Anterior Descending Artery or LAD that feeds the front and biggest portion of the heart. Two of the basic principles of *The Art of Heart Healing* are that the left side of the heart is concerned with relationships and the ventricle, or bottom part of the heart, represents giving. In an anterior MI, the greatest impact is to the left ventricle and represents how you give to yourself and others through relationships. The nature of a healthy relationship is a balance of give and take.

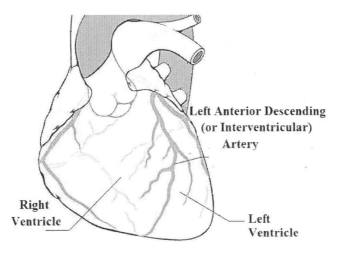

Source of Illustration: Coronary pdf: Patrick J Lynch, Medical Illustrator, derivative work: Fred the Oyster (talk), adaption and further labeling: Mikael Haggstrom

You've heard the term "leading with your heart." A heart attack involving the anterior wall highlights how you present yourself to the world through relationships. Are you forthcoming (upfront) with your feelings, or do you stop short of what your heart wants to feel. We all get guidance from our own hearts, but often we dismiss it as insignificant or even selfish. When you aren't true to your heart, it can affect relationships negatively and can show up as resentment, anger or frustration, and this stresses the system. It affects how you view yourself, others, and the world. The key to opening the door to vibrant circulation is to be in alignment with your heart by acknowledging those nudges from the heart. Be completely honest with yourself about your feelings around your relationships with your family and friends. "Heartfelt" feelings are a signal to pay attention. Making changes in your day-to-day interactions in accordance to heart guidance changes feelings and changes the very energy of your heart. This allows for alignment with your heart, increases flow and results in better performance.

Remember physical heart pain represents a starving heart. The flow to your heart stops short when you stop short of acknowledging and then acting on your true feelings. Problems here reflect your heart's desire to lead with compassion for yourself and others in the daily give and take of relationships while being true to who you are. If this desire is not fulfilled, your heart is not nourished and withers.

For example, I had a client who was diagnosed through a heart catheterization to have a 40% blockage of his LAD. He is a very giving person and has a very loving relationship with his wife of many years. He saw his job in this life was to be a support to his wife in all ways. This is a very noble view. The problem arises when his diligence in seeing that her wishes are met in every way compromises his own heart's desire to attend to his particular needs. Sometimes we are so focused on taking care of others and making sure their lives are complete, we forget to tune into our own hearts and tend to our garden to promote growth on our personal path.

Inferior MI

In the world of *The Art of Heart-Healing*, the right side of the heart reflects self-love. The Right Coronary Artery feeds primarily the right side and lower part of the heart. A heart attack that involves the RCA and affects this area is called an Inferior MI. This is another condition that is intuitively named. The term not only describes the location of the damage to the heart but also implies how we see ourselves: inferior, not enough, or not good enough. One way to compensate for these feelings may be to try to always be "right." Practice relinquishing the need to be right by realizing no one has all the answers to everything all the time. Would you rather be right or would you rather be happy?

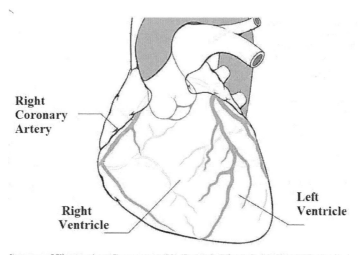

Right Coronary Artery

Right Ventricle

Left Ventricle

Source of Illustration:Coronary pdf: Patrick J Lynch, Medical Illustrator, derivative work: Fred the Oyster (talk), adaption and further labeling: Mikael Haggstrom

Coronary artery disease involving the right side of the heart is an opportunity to explore why we have feelings of "not being enough." Are they a result of well-meaning yet misguided parents whose praise we relied on to tell us how we were doing in life, but who never actually gave us the praise we needed? Withholding praise may have been to motivate us to do more, but instead set the tone as to how we talk to ourselves. This is not a call to blame parents; they parented the way they were parented, but rather a call to consciousness. If you become conscious of the conversation you have with yourself, you may find you say things you would never say to others. Be kind to yourself. We all make mistakes --- that's how we learn.

Posterior MI and Lateral MI

This can involve branches of the Left Coronary Artery (Circumflex Artery) or the Right Coronary Artery (Posterior Descending Artery). These are the arteries that feed the side and back areas of the heart so the damage is to the lateral wall or to the posterior wall. Energetically speaking, this is caused by pain that we've chosen to ignore, bury, keep secret or put aside or behind us. The discord of these events may or may not be in our awareness; nonetheless, it hasn't been dealt with. The clue to recognizing an area of your life that needs attention is a feeling of uneasiness or even pain when this part of your life comes to mind. This is graphically described by the phrase "smile though your heart is breaking." Pushing away ill feelings only magnifies them. Go through the past not around it. You don't need to dwell on it. If there is something about it that bothers you, acknowledge it and let some light shine on it. Being unwilling "to go there" inhibits full access to areas of your heart, and thus, decreasing flow to those areas. A heart attack happens when you have starved heart muscle, cut off from the whole. Become enlightened by your experiences. See the lesson and or the blessing in it rather than trying to cut yourself off from the experience by denying its existence. Find the treasure within.

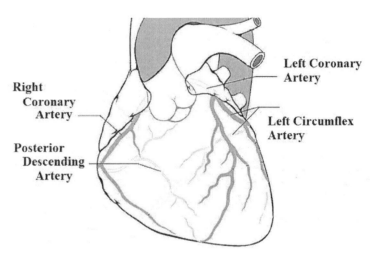

Source of Ilustration:Coronary pdf: Patrick J Lynch, Medical Illustrator, derivative work: Fred the Oyster (talk), adaption and further labeling: Mikael Haggstrom

Energetics of Dysrhythmias

Dysrhythmias are abnormal rhythms initiated by impulses that start the action of the heart and originate in the heart muscle outside the S.A. (Sino Auricular) node. The Sino Auricular node is the source of the inherent pacemaker of the heart and is located in the right upper heart.

Receiving is a function of the upper part of the heart or atrium where the impulse of the heart is located. The activation impulse then moves down to the ventricles, the bottom part of the heart that represents giving. When the impulse isn't initiated by the source, the synchronization between the receiving and giving chambers is lost and chaos ensues. We are taught it is more blessed to give than to receive which is only half the truth. The complete cycle involves receiving in order to have something to give.

The heart whose natural inclination is to follow the source is confused by the lack of direction of the random, unsynchronized impulses and has difficulty responding in an organized fashion. Energetically speaking, the natural order of things has been taken over by thought. Thoughts may become unaligned with the heart's inherent propensity toward simplistic solutions. Our thoughts and self-talk can derail the order of things and promote an imbalance in giving and receiving that obstructs flow. The electrical system of the heart is what synchronizes the action of the heart. Thoughts and negative self-talk can get in the way of synchronization.

The solution is to get our thoughts back in sync with the natural order of the universe. Most of us are consumed with thinking. We're taught you have to think of a solution, when in truth, the wisdom of the universe can be heard only in silence --- the silence in your mind. The silence is found between thoughts, and that is where total peace is accessed and self-acceptance follows. Self-acceptance is the antidote for over-thinking and obstructed flow. Through silence – such as meditation, or just focusing on your breath -- you can get in tune with the rhythm of the universe and allow your personal heart to entrain with the rhythm of the Universal Heart and unconditional love.

The more I learn about energy, the more I see how areas of my nursing career coincide with what I am learning in the world of energy. For instance, when I worked at Stanford in the 80's they had a very progressive dysrhythmia unit. We used temporary pacemakers that had the ability to pace at 300 beats/min. If a patient was in a very rapid rhythm that was life threatening, we would momentarily turn up the pacemaker to the rate that matched their heart rate to capture their rhythm, and then turn down the pacemaker to a normal rate and their heart rhythm would follow. This, in energy terms I have since learned, is entrainment.

Through silence you too can get in tuned with the rhythm of the Universe and allow your heart to entrain with the rhythm of the Universal Heart. Entrained with the Universal Heart, you will be in touch with endless creative potential.

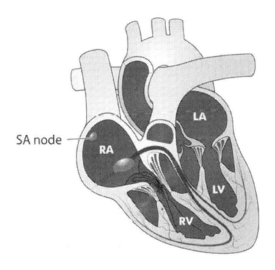

ILLUSTRATION OF:
SA (SINOAURICULAR) NODE

Palpitations

If the symptom of palpitations are present (they feel like "missed beats") that is a clue to explore the feeling of your heart's discontent. This is an opportunity to explore what you feel is "missing" in your life. Sometimes we have huge expectations in our lives. Occasionally they are expectations of others but often, when distilled, they are expectations of us. As I touched on earlier, self acceptance goes a long way in creating inner peace and allowing for flow. When we accept we have done our best with the knowledge and information we had at the time, we are much more able to forgive ourselves for perceived errors and obtain awareness of the growth we gained from our life situation.

Tachycardia

Tachycardia means to have a rapid heart rate. As established before, when the electrical system of the heart is in order, the rhythm is in sync with a natural order. When tachycardia or a very rapid heart rate is present, thoughts have derailed the process. Tachycardia can be likened to a runaway train, hence a "runaway-heart." The question you might ask is "what am I running away from?" Your heart is in sync with your runaway thoughts rather than your peaceful, all-knowing heart.

Tachycardia is an out-of-control feeling and results from going in a different direction than your heart's desire is directing you to go; in other words, not "following your heart." There is the addition of not feeling at peace and a sense of needing to tightly control events and people in our lives in order to know what to expect and thus, feel safe.

Awareness of behavior and its physical consequences is the first step in changing behavior and the end result. Take a few minutes to have awareness of what you are thinking when you feel your heart is "running away." Thoughts can be redirected to a more positive frame. This is the heart's natural state. It takes vigilance and practice but the results are lasting. You will recognize the heart's natural state by the inner feeling of "all is well" that follows.

Ventricular Tachycardia

As explained, a fast heart beat is like a runaway train. In ventricular tachycardia, the impulses that run the heart originate in the ventricles or giving part of the heart. This pacesetting focus is far away from the original source (intrinsic wisdom) and is traveling rapidly unsynchronized with the rest of the heart (the atria or receiving part). When this happens, the ventricle can't pause long enough to fully fill itself to expand and produce enough outflow to nourish itself or the rest of the body. This action of the ventricles is unsynchronized with the whole heart and the spirit of cooperation (rather than competition) is in jeopardy. This lack of cooperation can become so profound that the independent action of the heart is unable to sustain itself and ultimately the entire system. When this unsynchronized, uncooperative, independent action from the whole becomes so pronounced that chaos ensues, the rhythm of the heart deteriorates to ventricular fibrillation. In this state the result is an ineffective spasmodic motion of the ventricles, and the output is so compromised as to not be compatible with life.

This is representative of how you are conducting your life. Find time to focus on connecting with nature through intentional walks. Observing nature in your surroundings is helpful in regaining a sense of order and cooperation. Nature's way is the antithesis of competition; it is an all-encompassing, cooperative process that always seeks balance. Give to others from a place of desiring to be of service rather than out of duty; recognizing you are also giving yourself the gift of service.

Atrial or Supraventricular Tachycardia

In atrial or supraventricular tachycardia, instead of a single focus from the command center of the heart, there are one or more random impulses that originate in the upper chambers of the heart. The SA node is known as the heart's natural pacemaker and is in the receiving part of the heart. You want to receive from one source -- the natural source. The natural source is the field where all creative potential resides and is found in the stillness between thoughts accessible through quiet, harmonious heart space. If your mind is really busy, it is difficult to receive a signal from the intrinsic source. Instead the heart is directed by a single random signal or many random signals and is off and running. Quiet your mind to receive one signal. Allow your heart rather than your head to steer your life.

In atrial tachycardia, the runaway rhythm originates in the receiving chambers or atria. This is generally considered a less life threatening tachycardia than ventricular tachycardia. However this too is an impulse that has the trait of originating outside the original pacesetting source. Just as in a rhythm that originates in the ventricles, if the pace is rapid enough, it does not allow enough fill time for the giving chambers or ventricles and output is insufficient to nourish itself and others.

So in tachycardia, whether it's ventricular or atrial in origin, if the pace is rapid enough, the cardiac output isn't sufficient enough to be effective. The impulse is a runaway impulse that occurs without regard for the synchronization of the whole heart. When this occurs the heart's wisdom of cooperation in its parts, intricately designed to sustain itself and ultimately the entire system, is lost. When the focus of our thoughts isn't source driven or heart driven and in cooperation rather than in competition with the whole, the result is an insufficient output.

Atrial Fibrillation

Many of us don't know how to receive very well. We've established that normally there is a strong impulse from the sinus node that lives in the atrium or receiving part of the heart and initiates the heartbeat. In atrial fibrillation, there is no single strong impulse but many small, weak, randomly produced impulses that bombard the ventricles or giving chambers of the heart. The heart is confused and doesn't know which one to respond to or if to respond at all. If we rarely or never put ourselves in a position of receiving, we have no point of reference as to what it feels like to receive. Then we have multiple random impulses to give more and never feeling like we give enough.

Explore your motive for giving. Give from an authentic source of giving not from a place of giving to get. Set your intention to have a strong focus on receiving from a place of authenticity and imagine what that looks like as it runs through the giving part of your heart -- the ventricles –the main pumping section of your heart. See the clear circuit of receiving through your heart – the atrium or top part of your heart - so you have a strong impulse to give authentically from your heart.

I have a good friend who has developed atrial fibrillation. She grew up the oldest child in an unstable family where her father (whom she adored) was an alcoholic, and her mother, with three children, was always overwhelmed. She felt very unsafe and compensated by taking on the role of protector. As a child in order to control her environment, she tried to control all circumstances to keep her family safe. Exerting this kind of energy outward takes a lot of vigilance and effort.

This has carried over to adulthood and has become part of her fabric of being. If traveling in a car, she always drives because she gets motion sickness if riding. Unconsciously, moving her energy outside the bounds she has set for herself is so unfamiliar it causes physical symptoms of motion sickness. This is a metaphor for her life. Life is too scary and out of control if she's not the driver.

In truth, we are never the driver, we only think we are. The less complicated and truly effective way to live is to set things in motion and ride the wave --- to let go and let God! When we're always pushing it stops the flow. Plus, we are unable to receive when energy is being forcefully exerted to try to make things happen in a certain way. This is when we feel pressure. To be in the flow of the universe feels relaxed, able to respond to the next cue. Being unable to receive obstructs flow. When the flow of energy is decreased, it becomes dense and can solidify in the physical. The friend I mentioned has not only developed atrial fibrillation, but also kidney stones and gallstones.

Bradycardia

Bradycardia is defined in adults as a heart rate less than sixty beats per minute. This may or may not be a problem. If cardiac output (the amount of blood pumped by the heart) is not affected by this slow rate, there is no physiologic effect. I have found that people with a slow heart rate are very methodical. They consider every angle before acting. If the methodical process is such that it inhibits action, then output is affected and physical symptoms such as low blood pressure appear.

Long distance runners often have slow heart rates. It is a result of a strong heart. Their heart muscle is so strong that it takes fewer cycles to produce the same output as a weaker heart muscle. Metaphorically, they are continually putting one foot in front of the other moving forward. This creates inner power and is reflected in their hearts ability to produce.

In non athletes if a slow heart rate (bradycardia) is present, the impetus is slow. Since the impetus is slow, the flow may be slow and the output may be low. This can affect the nourishment of all systems of the body. Energetically, when we aren't listening to our heart's desire and staying in the flow of life, our work in the world is affected. Momentum is inhibited. In severe cases of low cardiac output (which corresponds to low work output) the blood flow to the brain may be diminished enough that unconsciousness can literally be the result. This represents our level of awareness of the problem. It indicates it is not on a conscious level and is a wakeup call.

Heart Block

A different category of an abnormally slow heart rate or bradycardia is Heart Block. This is a condition where the S.A. node impulse is not conducted through the heart muscle to contract the ventricles and circulate blood through the body. The impulse takes the path of least resistance through the electrical conduction system that is set up in the heart. If there is resistance in that pathway, the conduction is blocked and can't happen. In Heart Block, the impulse from the internal pacemaker to the heart is random, nonexistent, or it may exist, but is not conducted by the heart muscle. Since the heart is conducted by the impulse from the source, when the flow of conduction is hampered or nonexistent, the impulse to conduct our lives is hampered or, in severe cases, even nonexistent.

Just as the conductor conducts a symphony, the SA node conducts the symphony of the heart. If the members of the symphony aren't paying attention to the conductor, the parts aren't synchronized; and beautiful music is not the result. So it is with our heart. If our hearts aren't attuned to the conductor, the symphony of our heart is not played in a pleasing melodious way. Our hearts aren't conducted by the master impulse. Output is not on course, low, or nonexistent.

Pay attention to the synchronicities of life; act on the impulses generated by your heart and life will flow. Having resistance to these impulses inhibits flow and the symphony of life is literally out of tune.

With Heart Block there is resistance in the pathway of electrical conduction, and the impulse is blocked because there is a sense of decreased flow. Our goal is to change and increase the energy flow by repeated repatterning through awareness and taking guided action.

Junctional Rhythm

A junctional rhythm is one that is initiated by the AV (atrioventricular) node that is located between the atrium and ventricle, the receiving and giving chambers. This is usually a slow rhythm that automatically takes over if the normal heart rhythm is too slow. In terms of energy, if the natural pacemaker rhythm is slow to respond or totally obstructed by resistance in the pathway to conduction, a secondary pacemaker with a faster pace takes over to compensate for low output. Again, this is an opportunity to take a deep look at the initiation and direction of the guidance of your heart that can be accessed through stillness and a willingness to be completely honest with yourself about your feelings.

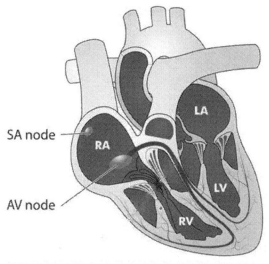

ILLUSTRATION OF:
AV (ATRIOVENTRICULAR) NODE

Often pacemakers are implanted to compensate for slow or nonexistent impulses from the natural pacemaker or SA node. These can be lifesaving. They are set to take over when your own intrinsic rhythm is too slow to effectively pump blood to your heart muscle and the rest of your body. To generate a heart-starting impulse from your own heart's desire is optimal. If you have a pacemaker, as you tune into your own heart intelligence and respond from that intrinsic knowing, you may find your own heart taking over and your artificial generator will need to respond less often.

Diseases of the Valves

There are generally two main problems that involve heart valves, stenosis and regurgitation. Stenosis is a narrowed valve opening while regurgitation has to do with a valve leaking. The most common valves involved are on the left side of the heart. The mitral valve is located between the two left chambers of the heart, and the aortic valve is the valve between the left ventricle and the aorta. The aorta is the large vessel that carries oxygenated blood from the left ventricle and branches off into the coronary arteries. The coronary arteries feed the heart itself and the main aorta supplies nourishment to the entire body. *The Art of Heart Healing* defines the association of the left side of the heart energetically with relationship love.

<u>Regurgitation</u>

Regurgitation is a term used to describe what occurs when a valve doesn't close effectively. The valve is the gatekeeper. This closing action prevents a backflow of blood up into the chamber it is gate keeping. When regurgitation occurs, blood that should be pumped forward regurgitates back up into the heart. Another term for this condition is insufficiency because the valve doesn't close sufficiently to prevent a backward flow. It can't sufficiently keep the focus of forward flow from "going back there."

Are you continually "going back there" to replay, rehash, and regurgitate events you perceive as troubling, often hoping they will look differently and then feeling insufficient when this only seems to magnify the problem? Regurgitating and replaying an event in which you see yourself or someone else as insufficient only embeds this energy in the system and promotes a sense of being a "victim of circumstance." This can result in a feeling of powerlessness in a world of turmoil.

Because replaying events and emotions in your head reinforces and multiplies the negative energy, you must change the focus to achieve a different result. Monitor your thoughts. When you find yourself "going back there," make a choice to consciously change your focus. Retraining your mind retrains your emotional heart and subsequently your physical heart. This cuts the ties to the past and frees the heart of its emotional and physical limitations compromised by being bound to the past.

Stenosis

With a stenotic or narrowed valve, the blood is not able to be freely pumped to the receiving chamber or vessel. The gatekeeper (the valve) has held back and due to a lack of flow, forward movement is slowed and the contents become stagnant. The energy of the previous cardiac cycle is held onto. Energetically, it mingles with the past. It's important to release the past. It's not relevant to the new energy being circulated in the present. The uncirculated volume increases as unreleased blood mixes with the new oxygenated blood in the left side of the heart, and the pressure to release increases.

Stenosis refers to a choking of the natural flow. Take an honest look at the give and take in relationships. Are you able to flow with day to day interactions or do you keep score and withhold according to your perception of the worthiness of others. Ask yourself if others' actions are the criteria you use to determine if they are worthy to be the beneficiary of your approval. You must detach from the need to control others, stop keeping score; give and release. Let go of attempts to control mundane details of relationships and open to the flow of the present moment.

Mitral Regurgitation

The mitral valve is the gatekeeper between the receiving and giving chambers of the left side of the heart. When mitral regurgitation occurs, blood that should be pumped to the ventricle regurgitates back up into the atrium. This lowers the blood pressure and increases the work load of the left upper chamber, the atrium. Remember another term for this condition is mitral insufficiency. Explore the perception you have of your role in a situation that is disturbing to you. Be clear about what you feel you are receiving.

If you feel compromised in having your own needs met and what you receive from a relationship feels insufficient, the tendency is not to perform from a place of inner strength but rather from a place of ambivalence. This may result in feeling insufficient yourself. Even if you can't change your circumstances, you can change the perception of your circumstances. This change in perception will facilitate energy flow to the next stage without wishing you could take it back or feeling you are held back. Again, an honest look at your true feelings will reveal where those feelings come from.

Often the lack of forward movement is attributed to an interaction with someone else, and that may be a contributing factor. However, in the end, you are responsible for how you react to restrictions directed by others. You have a choice, even if it's only a choice in perception. This involves taking responsibility for all that occurs in your life. Moving to the next step without looking back and without second guessing yourself decreases your work load and frees you to be more productive. After you make a decision close the door to rethinking your choice.

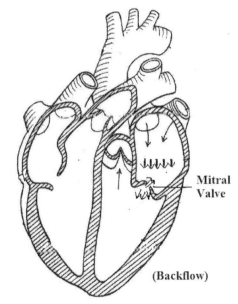

ILLUSTRATION OF:
MITRAL REGURGITATION

Aortic Regurgitation

In aortic regurgitation, blood leaks back into the left ventricle in between beats when the heart is resting. This blood is stagnant and, along with new blood that has entered from the upper chamber with the next beat, must be pumped out. The low output of blood to the body may result in symptoms of congestive heart failure, angina (chest pain), and low blood pressure. If you have these symptoms refer to those sections for more information on the components that result from this condition.

The aortic valve is the gatekeeper between the left ventricle and the aorta. The left ventricle has the largest capacity in terms of volume and work load of the heart. It is the giver to the heart itself and to the body. The aorta is the pathway to the heart muscle and is the bridge to the rest of the body. Again if you continually rethink every move before you make a final decision, clarity is lost; a clear decision to move forward is compromised and stagnation occurs. You not only see yourself as insufficient in terms of productivity in accomplishing in your own life but also in relationship with others.

This added volume causes the left ventricle to become enlarged and thickened. It is then less pliable, and output is lessened. As you dwell on feelings, they become a part of your fiber, and you may become overwhelmed and too immobilized to be productive. This state can be reflected in the function of your heart muscle. This immobility compounds your inability to be productive in a way that nourishes your own heart and that impacts your relationships. If your feelings are ignored or aren't recognized, you can't effectively act on your circumstances to navigate through the passivity to see your way out of a stagnant situation. This can build on itself and result in feelings of guilt and powerlessness.

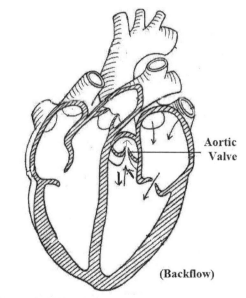

Aortic
Valve

(Backflow)

ILLUSTRATION OF:
AORTIC REGURGITATION

Mitral Stenosis

The mitral valve is the gatekeeper between the receiving chamber and the giving chamber on the relationship side of the heart. In mitral stenosis the gatekeeper prevents flow due to its inability to let go and open up. Explore your own feelings around how you view giving to others. Do you hold back fearing you'll say or do the wrong thing. The freedom to flow in everyday interactions comes from understanding that your past experiences don't dictate the outcome for today. When you hold back because of past memories, the contents of your offering becomes stagnant and only adds pressure to release the old ideas and move forward with fresh energy – a new way of seeing an old situation. Remember life is a constant flow, the past is done. When flow is hampered by thoughts that restrict movement, your ability to receive is impacted because you have retained energy that was designed to be given to the next stage of circulating energy. This holding back of circulating energy diminishes flow that is vital to nourish yourself and your relationships.

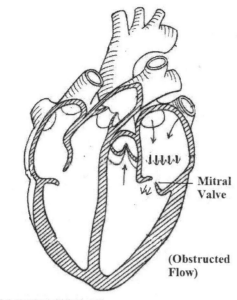

Mitral
Valve

(Obstructed
Flow)

ILLUSTRATION OF:
MITRAL STENOSIS

Aortic Stenosis

The aortic valve is the gatekeeper between the left ventricle, the giving chamber and the aorta, the large vessel that distributes new vitality to the heart itself and the entire body. With aortic stenosis, the gatekeeper has created a narrowed opening that restricts the opportunity for the hearts contents to be circulated to feed itself and others. This may be a slight restriction or may progress to the stage that greatly diminishes the flow of life. With severe restrictions the backup of uncirculated energy becomes so great that the pressure on the giver results in a thickened skin. In the medical world, when the wall of the ventricle is thickened, it is said the heart is less compliant. The pump itself is compromised when less compliant and the ability to flow what is in your heart to give is greatly diminished. This affects how you are in the world in terms of giving to your own heart's need and subsequently impedes your ability to give to others because you are out of touch with that desire. This affects all areas of life including relationships. The job of life can seem so full of obstacles that it feels as if you are swimming upstream and all joy is lost. This results in less output or satisfaction and less nourishment of yourself and others.

Aortic Stenosis is energetically preceded by a holding back action around one's deepest desires. Learn to listen for clues from your heart about what you truly desire. If you have an idea about what might make you happy, go with it. Lessen your grip on thinking about how you need to give, and focus on how you want to give. Give from a place of ease rather than "shoulds." Put your hand over your heart and set the intention to give deeply from the well of your being to yourself and others.

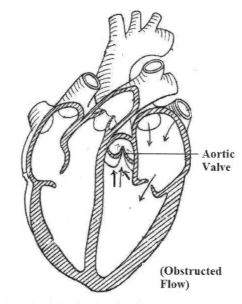

Aortic
Valve

(Obstructed
Flow)

ILLUSTRATION OF:
AORTIC STENOSIS

Mitral Valve Prolapse

A separate valve problem is Mitral Valve Prolapse, the most frequently diagnosed heart valve problem. It most commonly affects females and tends to run in families. The mitral valve leaflets are more elastic that normal and stretch back up into the left upper chamber when the left lower chamber contracts. The place to look for an understanding of the feelings involved is your perception of what you receive in a relationship in proportion to what you give. The symptoms include rapid or irregular heartbeat. Energetically, this indicates an erratic feeling about a relationship and is based on the perception of being "let down." Resentment surfaces surrounding the realization, "I've taken care of you; where are you when I need you?"

Mitral valve prolapse is also associated with a feeling of not belonging. This can be on all levels - spiritually, physically, and emotionally. Trying to "fit in" can foster giving from a feeling of obligation rather than from your heart. This originates from a belief that you should be a certain way or do certain things in order for others to accept or love you. In mitral valve prolapse, the valve is so elastic that the leaflets of the valve stretch back up into the atrium or receiving chamber. Do you bend over backwards in an attempt to feel worthy of receiving in a relationship? This can result in a feeling of self-sacrifice and when someone doesn't reciprocate or appreciate your sacrifice, you may feel "let down." To remedy this, know that it's in your best interest (as well as everyone else's) to give only when your heart truly desires to do so rather than being driven by feelings of obligation.

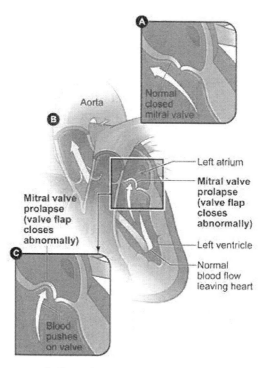

Source of Illustration: National Heart, Lung, and Blood Institute; National Institutes of Health

Congestive Heart Failure

In congestive heart failure the heart is overloaded or burdened due to the diminished amount of blood pumped to meet the needs of the body and the needs of the heart itself. The result is fluid retention in the tissues. Again, these conditions are intuitively described when referenced by the medical community. If someone has congestive heart failure it is said "they are in failure" or "overloaded." The reference is to failure of the heart muscle due to diminished contractility and an overload of fluid accumulated in the heart and lungs because of reduced cardiac output - that is, the amount of blood pumped out by the left ventricle. Because diminished heart function results in reduced cardiac output this condition is referred to as "low output state."

These phrases completely embody what is occurring emotionally. Frequently you have taken on responsibilities outside your range of effectiveness. This is not a reflection on your capability, although that is how it is internalized. They are burdens that aren't yours to bear, and the extent to which you involve yourself becomes overwhelming. Your heart feels heavy, bogged down, and overloaded. Feeling as though you have failed either yourself or someone else, the perceived burden of the effort to rectify this situation (or even where to start) is immobilizing and low output results.

Congestive heart failure can occur on both sides of the heart and energetically the cause is different. Right sided heart failure indicates diminished vitality that results from carrying the burden of self failure and produces a feeling of "heavy heartedness." This feeling of heaviness can be lessened by "lightening" your heart; that is, by lifting the burden of self-blame or self-criticism and by seeing challenges as opportunities to grow.

Left sided heart failure also stems from a feeling of "heavy heartedness," but this diminished vitality has its roots in the burden of failure associated with relationships. The heaviness produced by these feelings comes about from the decreased energy put into a relationship because the amount of effort required for interaction seems overwhelming. This leads to stagnation in your own vitality and negatively impacts your output to the world.

Both types of heart failure can produce shortness of breath which reflects a sense of not being true to yourself. Ask what is it you want to do not only in life, but in this moment. Be perfectly honest with your response even if you think it's not acceptable or doable. Often just taking this first step of acknowledging desires is dismissed because the uncertainty of how change might look is simply too scary. You don't have to make huge changes and sometimes skipping steps can be too big a leap to be comfortable. The first step is simply to acknowledge what isn't working, and then take a small step toward changing that.

A common symptom of congestive heart failure is swelling of the feet and legs. Look to areas in your life where you don't feel supported. If there are times when you feel all alone there are solutions. Often those who could help you aren't aware of your feelings. Be up front with what you need. If you know that people close to you aren't available for whatever reason, ask those you know will be responsive. Again rather than seeing yourself as a victim of circumstance, change the circumstance. In this age of instant communication, there is immediate access to the help you need, but you have to be willing to see the possibilities; ask and then be willing to receive.

From a spiritual point of view, feeling unsupported is an opportunity to look at emotions around your belief in energy forces outside the tangible world available through prayer or meditation. Feeling connected to nature, an omnipotent force such as God and angels, or whatever your belief system embraces is paramount in creating the feeling you are not alone. This can be challenging for some because it involves the element of trust. Noticing and acknowledging positive energy influences around a troubling situation goes a long way in creating more synchronistic events and builds trust around the idea you are not alone.

Hypertension

Blood pressure is the measure of pressure in the blood vessels during systole (contraction of the heart) and diastole (relaxation of the heart). The top number of a blood pressure reading represents pressure exerted on arteries during systole, and the bottom number of a reading represents the pressure exerted during diastole. These numbers are elevated in high blood pressure. The causes of high blood pressure may include some hormonal abnormalities and arteriosclerosis (diseased arteries).

Energetically the increased pressure symbolized by high blood pressure is twofold. It represents the increased pressure you put on yourself to do more – never satisfied, always pushing, and it also represents the resistance to seeing things differently to allow for changes in behavior.

There is a direct correlation between the amount of resistance in the circulatory system and the pressure exerted on the vessels of the body measured by blood pressure. That is, if there is increased systemic vascular resistance due to narrowed vessels caused by diseased arteries or the release of stress hormones, blood pressure is elevated. The energetic translation is the more resistance there is to acknowledging and looking at situations that aren't working or burying feelings, especially those of anger, resentment, or powerlessness, the more rigid and inflexible you become to changing your circumstances.

When this happens, your view of things gets narrower and narrower, and it becomes more and more difficult to see a way out of your current state of being. The higher the pressure in the arteries, the more inflexible they are and the narrower they become which only increases the pressure, and it's a continuous cycle. The materialization of this energy in the circulatory system is rigidity and narrowing in the arteries and is known as arteriosclerosis or hardening of the arteries. This condition inhibits flow. The path of least resistance is staying in the flow -- allowing events of your life to flow rather than always "pushing the river."

As the internal pressure increases for us to be in integrity, so does the blood pressure. To acknowledge true feelings brings them into conscious awareness. When you bring hidden or buried emotions to light, you come into integrity.

Often a pattern of needing to have things in a certain order and resistance to seeing any other way, are set early in life. It can be a response to a need to feel safe. My own experience is a prime example of how early events can influence responses to life situations and set up a pattern of narrow thinking in an attempt to feel safe. As a child growing up in an alcoholic family where I had little say about our chaotic home environment, it has been my quest in life to have order. That, for me, meant not only feeling responsible for my own actions but a very real feeling of responsibility for everyone else. This manifested in relationships with my family as well as in the work place. In Critical Care, I not only felt responsible for the well-being of the patient to whom I was assigned, but for the well-being of all the patients in the unit along with their families and even the other nurses I worked with. As you can imagine, this was a daunting assignment. I have come to realize this is a result of not accepting myself. When I accept myself, I am free to accept everyone else and honor their ability to handle situations that are theirs to handle.

When self acceptance is incomplete (the microcosmic view), it expands to not accepting others and then extends to the world (the macrocosmic view). There is a tendency to continually push to make things happen. The focus becomes "willing things done" which ultimately is an outward motion of energy or pushing things away rather than accepting that there is some divine order that allows for the possibility of a bigger picture. When you open yourself to acceptance, you open the door to receiving. To energetically enhance self acceptance, have the intention to allow yourself to be open to receive. It is an ongoing process, but being mindful of behavior is huge in changing it.

The constant activity of pushing to do more is an activity of the head not the heart. This increased activity to produce from the mind increases pressure in the head as well as the rest of the body, and headaches may be present in high blood pressure. If headaches are present, this adds the component of being "in your head" while trying to solve problems and not looking to be spiritually and emotionally guided through your heart.

Relaxing into situations and allowing things to flow reduces the pressure from constant mental activity and restores the normal pressure in all the body including the head. An intention to be heart-centered rather than head-centered is paramount in eliminating high blood pressure and accompanying head pain. Again this is accomplished through an awareness of your true desires and acting on those rather than what you "think" you should do.

With high blood pressure, sometimes hormonal messengers that regulate the blood pressure are abnormal. This is a result of stress. Stress is a comprehensive category of events that puts a strain on the system. When released, hormones may trigger symptoms of stress such as high blood pressure. Look to hidden messages from your family and how that influenced you to avoid conflict in order to keep the peace. This concept was first introduced to me by Meredith Young Sowers at Stillpoint.

Sometimes parents focused on one thing but the underlying message was something else. For example as a young woman I was encouraged to look a certain way and act a certain way. Much emphasis was put on outward appearance and what the neighbors would think. The hidden message was: Your worth is determined by how you look on the outside not by who you are on the inside. The message went even further than that: Who you are is not enough. I often complied with the established ways of being to keep the peace even though deep down I didn't agree.

As an adult the pressure becomes more intense to follow your heart in what you know to be in integrity with who you are. It is important to listen to your inner guidance and respond accordingly to relieve that pressure. Awareness is the first step in bringing your body back to energetic balance. Physical activity such as stretching exercises or yoga increases the flexibility of the body and translates into flexibility of the mind.

Cardiomyopathy

I have a particular interest in cardiomyopathy. Any heart disease can be challenging but this disease, in my experience, can be devastating. I worked at Stanford Medical Center Hospital for six years in the 1980's. This hospital performed some of the early heart transplants. I took care of many young people who died waiting for heart transplants, but one young man particularly stands out in my memory. His boggy heart condition was attributed to a reaction to the many vaccines he was required to take as a soldier. Often the only hope offered for people with severe cardiomyopathy is a heart transplant, but for him the wait was too long. In retrospect, exploring the feelings around these events in his life may have paved the way to heart changing energy. He and many others have inspired me to find another solution to regenerate diseased heart muscle. I find the growing awareness of both the heart's intrinsic nervous system and the heart's connection to its own healing energy field very exciting!

Cardiomyopathy literally means "disease of the heart muscle". This results in poor pump action and low output state. The term Global Hypokinesis is given to the generalized poor contractility of the heart. The main symptom is congestive heart failure. As in the chapter on congestive heart failure, this malady has its energetic roots in failure due to being burdened and overloaded. Because this affects the whole heart rather than a specific part, it is termed global. Just as this is a global condition of the heart, it can ultimately become a global condition of the body and affect other organs because all parts rely on the heart to supply them with nourished blood. The underlying physiology for cardiomyopathy may be the result of a viral infection, coronary artery disease, alcohol ingestion, post partum (after having a baby) or idiopathic which means the cause is unknown.

In cardiomyopathy the heart's poor contractility results in dilation due to poor pump action, and its inability to express blood due to diminished action. The heart holds onto that which is ready to be expressed, and this inhibits its ability to create a fully productive next cycle. The heart becomes overwhelmed with the increased work load, and failure is the result. The heart literally becomes heavy, weighted down with excess fluid and poorly functioning heart muscle.

A heavy heart is often used to describe someone in grief. Cardiomyopathy is global grief. The global part of the heart references your connection to the rest of the world – the unity of all things. Cardiomyopathy is global grief over not being able to wholeheartedly feel the loving vibration of the One Heart which connects us all in the web of life.

When we are in grief, there is often an inability to recognize the heart's connectedness to a universal consciousness that embodies the wisdom of divine order and inspires creation that feeds the soul. Without this connection we can become out of touch with the rhythm of life, and the rhythm that is our heart. The natural order directs the mind to cooperate with the heart, not compete. When the mind and heart are in a harmonious state, the mind does not work in opposition to the heart. In the process of cardiomyopathy, the role of the mind and the heart may become confused, and the mind can take over the role of the heart because of the heart's weakened state.

Grief occurs when a bond to something we were attached to feels broken, and a sense of emptiness takes its place. Commonly this is intuitively referred to as "losing heart." Because you have lost heart, there is a shift in roles (mind overrules heart) and a shift in perception. The perception of the mind is that this bond was what made you feel not alone and gave your life purpose - a reason to live. Your heart knows that you are never alone for you are irrevocably connected to all that is. When the mind and the heart are in conflict, apathy of the heart may ensue --- even down to the apathy of the heart muscle to contract. The stimulus to produce action is blocked. Reawakening that connection to the energy of wholeness is the key to reawakening the energy of the heart muscle. This is accomplished through awareness and intention. Shift the focus of power from your mind to your heart. This is the shift in consciousness from victim to creator.

Flow in the heart is measured by cardiac output. The amount of flow is determined by pressure over resistance. The degree you are in the flow is determined by the pressure generated by your heart's desire compared to the resistance generated in the system intended to circulate the output. Resistance may be met in the lungs as the blood passes through to be oxygenated. This impairs inspiration which is the medical term for the in-breath. This determines the quality and quantity of what you take in to nourish your heart and body not only physically but spiritually. The term inspiration can also refer to divine influence, so this is cause and effect defined by one word. Your inspiration affects your inspiration. That is: the quality of your breath influences the quality of your creative thought, your inner wisdom.

Resistance may be met not only in the lungs but also throughout the vascular system of the body. This is referred to as total peripheral resistance. This resistance is one of the factors that determines flow and if high, hampers circulation. In cardiomyopathy, because the output of the heart is diminished, one of the treatments is to relax the arterial blood vessels of the body with medication to lower systemic vascular resistance. Remember we said one of the main symptoms of cardiomyopathy is congestive heart failure, and in CHF the heart is overloaded or burdened. Reducing systemic vascular resistance allows the heart not to have to work as hard to pump blood to the body and itself. The heart muscle is in a state of "I can't do it anymore." This is a good time to release the idea that, "I am responsible for making everything in my life and other's lives happen even though my heart isn't in it." It's time to simply allow flow.

The diminished flow in cardiomyopathy is characterized by a boggy heart. Regardless of the underlying cause of cardiomyopathy, it is the body's attacks on itself as a result of the mind's perception of self failure. Energetically, self-blame perpetuates a loss of power to make choices that propel you forward and instead bogs down the workings of the heart.

A reduction in the power of the heart is perpetuated by reluctance to being true to the singing of your "heart song." When your heart is in tune with your true self, it is free to sing your heart song. Your heart song is the passion that fulfills your heart's desire to accomplish your life plan. Recognizing and pursuing your passion or heart song keeps your heart in rhythm with your life's purpose.

Your heart song is what you came to give to others in order to heal that in yourself. What you extend to others is strengthened in you. Your heart is a muscle. Just as the muscle in your arm is strengthened if you extend it to help someone up, the more you extend your heart in service, the stronger it becomes. The louder you sing your heart song, the more people it reaches and the more it reverberates in you.

Identifying your heart song can take some detective work. Noticing what you do in your life that animates you, the theme of the movies you watch, the books you read, what activities you gravitate towards in your spare time, and what subject lights you up when you're engaged in conversation can all be clues about what your heart desires.

My own personal journey of self discovery has been ongoing as I suspect it is in most people. I didn't just wake up one morning knowing what I wanted to do to make my heart happy. However, I did look back on my life at one point in my fifties and realized that my primary focus of interest and learning had always been heart related. Not only had my career focus been on heart health, but I had many experiences of the heart (a tumultuous childhood, divorce, death of a spouse) that gave me a personal education of the feelings involved and helped prepare me for this work. I began noticing how passionate I felt every time the subject of hearts came up. That was my first awareness that heart health as it relates to the energy of emotion might be my passion and gave me a clue to the purpose I had set for myself in this life. So think about what "lights you up" and how the work in your life up to now relates to that passionate feeling for clues to your "heart song."

Golden Grid Healing

Cardiomyopathy is a global condition of depleted energy of the heart that weakens the structure. Golden Grid Healing is a short exercise designed to energize your heart. It has become a very important tool for me. I use it with clients to help them heal an emotion or condition by fusing a golden grid with their heart muscle. I first saw this golden grid many years ago when I was conducting a healing on a diseased tree in my back yard. I knew it was a healing grid, but that's about all I knew. I have since used it to aid heart healing. I've come to realize it can be placed around something to be healed, such as a heart, or around the whole person or animal. The grid seems to contain information that accesses the healing power of oneness and makes it available for you to heal in all directions of time and on all levels of your being. The Golden Grid transitions you to a state of Grace to allow healing.

Golden Grid Exercise

Close your eyes and take an easy breath through your heart. This gets you in touch with your heart. Imagine a beautiful Golden Grid of light that gently surrounds you. It feels light yet strongly present as it envelops you and lifts you up to a higher state of presence. This golden mesh merges with your heart, and you see your heart become a radiant golden beacon of light. A beautiful yellow light forms at the base of your breast bone and has the strength of the glowing sun. This brilliant yellow light expands into and merges with the golden light of your heart reinforcing its strength. You feel the tension in your body ease as a warm glow envelops your entire body. You feel light and free as you absorb the glow from the Golden Grid, taking in only the information you need for your individual healing on your journey to wholeness. You have a growing sense of warmth, safety, inner power, and a feeling "all is well." When you're ready, open your eyes knowing the Golden Grid will stay in place until the work is complete.

Heartache and Grief

Heartache is a byproduct of grief and can affect the whole heart – giving, receiving, self love, and relationship love. Heartache is a result of a perceived loss. As humans we fill ourselves up with things outside ourselves such as jobs, relationships, status in life and when those things go for whatever reason death, divorce, job loss we suffer a feeling of loss. This perceived loss creates a void that cannot be filled no matter what we do - a loneliness that persists no matter how many people are around. This void fills with pain, and heartache is born.

Loss is created as a result of the mind's attachment to the way things were. You become familiar with the energy of others and the situations around those interactions and when that energy changes, the loss of familiarity is very unsettling. This shift in energy leaves a feeling of emptiness. It is a feeling of not being filled full no matter how much action you take. Action is an attempt to fill the void from the mind's perspective when in fact, the solution is an energetic shift from the mind to the heart. The heart knows that this attachment created by the mind was formed from the erroneous idea you can ever be separated from the whole. Heartache stems from a longing for wholeness. We all have a memory of wholeness no matter how distant. We long to remember (put together) the feeling of wholeness --- to fill the void.

As an example, I'll share my own experience of heartache. My significant other of twenty years, Terry, died suddenly at the age of fifty-three of heart disease while walking on his treadmill. Even though I was immensely sad, I put on my game face and went about life. My parents and sisters didn't want to see me in pain so when they asked how I was doing I'd say "fine" and hide the emptiness and sadness I really felt. In fact I wasn't even honest with myself about my emotions. In addition I tended to be really critical of myself for not being able to erase the loneliness. If I couldn't accept my own feelings, how could I expect others to accept my feelings? Now more than ever it's important to live in integrity. We used to think of that as not stealing or lying. At this time being in integrity extends even farther to include being perfectly honest with yourself about how you feel in all areas of your life.

I was still working in coronary care so a big part of my job was to care for fifty-three year old men with heart disease. Because I denied how I truly felt, I didn't recognize my own needs so I could not give to myself or ask for what I needed. I didn't know how to allow others to give to me. This greatly prolonged my grief process.

This way of thinking is an imbalance of the divine masculine and divine feminine energies. Having a balance of these energies in both men and women is optimal. The divine masculine energy creates doing and the divine feminine energy gives rise to receiving. I was so busy "doing" to avoid feeling what was painful that I couldn't stop long enough to receive from others who were willing to give to me. This widens the gap of feeling separate and heightens a sense of aloneness.

The other missing component in the healing process is acceptance that there is some larger plan at work, and all is in divine order. Instead I ran through my head constantly how, if this hadn't happened, things might have been different, and I knew for sure I would have been happier. These twinges of regret and "only ifs" are rooted in a sense of powerlessness rather than in trust that all is in divine order. This leap of faith to acceptance can be a really tall order when you are in pain. Now, when I look back I realize that if Terry and I continued together, my journey in the world of heart healing would have had many more obstacles because he did not embrace this work. His leaving the physical world had a hidden gift, even though at the time you would never have convinced me of that.

Even with great reluctance to move through this process, sometimes the universe gives you another opportunity to revisit and release grief through synchronicity. For me, this opportunity came several years after Terry's death. I had been doing energy work with a young man, twenty-three years old, through my hospice work. I had seen him every week for about three months before he passed on. His funeral was three days later, and I felt an overwhelming sadness. I was puzzled as to my reaction at the funeral when I could not quit crying until I realized it was the six-year anniversary of Terry's death. From this I learned that if you have not finished with the process of grief, somehow it will resurface. It is important to honor that.

A sudden loss such as the death of a loved can even precipitate a physiological event of the heart. This was described in a syndrome identified by doctors at Johns Hopkins in the New England Journal of Medicine in Feb just before Valentine's Day of 2005, called "broken heart syndrome." It is described as "stress cardiomyopathy" and the study found that emotional stress can cause severe but reversible dysfunction of the heart muscle that mimics a heart attack. [ii]

This wasn't a surprise to many associated with the care of heart patients. We often saw patients who could even verbalize that they had a "broken heart." The good news is we now know it's reversible if the patient's vital signs can be supported medically through the crisis. By that I mean there is medication to support low blood pressure or correct life threatening abnormal heart rhythms as well as procedures to enhance poorly functioning heart muscle during a crisis sustained by the heart. I encourage anyone with an acute potentially life threatening cardiac condition to take advantage of the extensive medical knowledge and treatment available. It truly saves lives.

There is no timetable to walk through grief to soothe heartache. The steps of grief can be compared to a house with many rooms for it has many facets and can be complicated. In this house of heartache, each room has many windows, the shades are drawn and the house is very dark. Sometimes you remain stuck in one room or move on to the next room without lifting all the shades, and it may seem as if this feeling of hopelessness will never change. Commonly this is referred to as "losing heart." You feel alone in the dark, separateness expands, and the void in your heart widens with pain. Pain and darkness are much denser than light and your heart goes from being lighthearted to heavy hearted.

As you shift the focus from mind-centered loss to heart-centered acceptance, you are able to raise the shades in the room one at a time to allow the light in. You are then free to move to the next room or the next stage. In time, you lift all the shades to the windows of your heart, and light fills the void replacing the darkness with hope. There is no schedule for moving through these rooms or steps of grieving, and everyone is different so be true to your own feelings. When you are not true to your feelings, you delay the process and can remain stuck in the energy of grief, just as I did. When this happens powerlessness can result.

Disempowerment impacts the energy power center of the body and weakens it. This power center runs most efficiently on clear power from within not the power you seek externally. That's why it is important to address your inner needs in order to move forward. This power center governs the muscles of the body and further explains how loss of power may literally affect your ability to move forward. The heart is a muscle. If the grief process is prolonged the actual myocardium or heart muscle may become malnourished. That is sometimes when heartache can progress to heart disease.

Physical movement can be an important part of grief recovery, but the word "exercise" is so off-putting when you're in grief. Your response might be, "How can I exercise when I can barely get out of bed?" Something as simple as walking strengthens your energy and stimulates your muscles, including the heart muscle. The act of walking symbolizes putting one foot in front of the other on the path of healing and hope for a brighter day.

Cholesterol

Cholesterol is found in the membrane of the cell and is a necessary component for its existence. It has many functions – one of which is cellular repair. Cholesterol is often misunderstood. It is a fat (lipid) manufactured by the liver and is seen as the enemy of the heart and blood vessels. It has even been given "sides" - good cholesterol and bad cholesterol. It's no wonder that we see it as something we need to fight. LDL (low density lipoprotein, also known as "bad" cholesterol) carries cholesterol to the cells and HDL (high density lipoprotein or so called "good" cholesterol) carries cholesterol back to the liver.

One cause of heart attacks is clogged arteries, secondary to plaque buildup. Why does plaque form? The tendency is to blame the circulation of too much "bad" cholesterol (LDL) in the system. A better question might be, "Why is so much LDL being supplied to the cells that compose the lining of the arteries?"

When there is inflammation in the arteries, this sets up a sequence of events that allows for repair of that artery. One such event is a call for increased production of cholesterol to be delivered to the inflamed site for repair. A more useful question than "How can I lower the production of bad cholesterol (LDL)?" might be, "How can I lower the inflammation in my arteries that requires increased production of LDL?" More specifically you might ask, "What is running my life that causes me irritation and sometimes even inflames me?"

If you have elevated cholesterol, the two points of focus by the medical profession are heredity and diet. Maybe we are missing the boat. Since we are all composed of energy, perhaps we should consider the energy we infuse our cells with through our thoughts and emotions. Just because we cannot see the energy of a thought or emotion, does not make them any less powerful. We can't see gravity or electricity, but we can see their effects.

I have had many clients come to me with the belief that their fate is sealed because of a genetic predisposition to high cholesterol. Through the groundbreaking work of cellular biologist Dr. Bruce Lipton, the old idea that a cell's behavior is determined merely by its genetic make-up has become obsolete. The notion that having a family history of increased cholesterol means you will inevitably have the same problem is also obsolete.

Dr. Lipton's work promotes the idea that cell behavior is determined by its environment created by beliefs rather than its genetic make-up. He teaches the membrane of the cell is the brain of the cell not the nucleus where the chromosomes are found. The protein receptors in the cell's membrane determine which molecules attach and enter the cell. LDL and HDL are lipoproteins – fats connected to proteins. Remember LDL stands for low density and HDL stands for high density. However, there are even variables of density within these two groups, and the cell determines which molecules it receives based on its environment. It stands to reason if the cell is in an environment that needs repair, more cholesterol will be circulated to be available to the cell.

This again points to the importance of the environment you create in your body with your thoughts and perceptions about yourself, your life and the world. Is it a view that ignites inflamed thoughts, or is it one that promotes thoughts that help decrease or alleviate disruptions that come your way?

Your job is to reduce the need for repair. To do that, become aware of the thoughts that are running in your mind. They are often ones you learned from your family of origin. The ideas passed down from generation to generation are more of a determinate of your physical state than the actual genes passed down. What you circulate in your life – through your thoughts and emotions -- determines what is circulated in your cells.

Now that we've looked at the heredity aspect let's focus on another cause of elevated cholesterol levels -- diet. Diet is very important. From the perspective of overall health (body and mind), the idea is to look at your diet not so much as anti-cholesterol, but rather from the point of engendering the desire to eat higher quality food.

In doing so, your biologic composition will also be higher quality. Remember that there have been a number of studies done on plants proving that they have a form of consciousness (see suggested reading). Wouldn't you rather eat foods that are raised in an environment of care and productiveness based on traditional methods that promote healthy plants and soil?

It is more important to concentrate on consuming the highest quality food attainable, than to just focus on lowering cholesterol. Your diet will reflect that intent and focusing on cholesterol is of less concern. Remember that quantum physics tells us without doubt that everything is energy of varying frequency. As we've talked about previously, your thoughts carry frequencies of energy, too. Having the intention to eat a high quality diet is a positive thought-form that is reflected in the food choices you make. This makes it easier to take actions in the best direction for your health. And of course, taking action is the most important step. Changing your diet can be daunting, but taking steps in that direction is empowering.

In Conclusion…

My motivation for exploring the emotions associated with heart disease was the frustration I felt as a nurse in educating patients about what to do to prevent another occurrence of heart disease. Often the conversation centered on life style changes such as diet, exercise, and smoking. These are the environmental changes we are all familiar with, but if you have a family history of heart disease, often you are told it is the luck of the genetic draw and that ultimately determines your fate no matter what you do.

As we shift our way of being from victims of life to creators of our personal life, there are many pioneers who have dedicated their work to establishing a new paradigm. Through the innovative work of cell biologist, Bruce Lipton, the old way of thinking that cellular behavior is determined by its genetic make-up has been challenged. He has shown that cellular behavior is determined by its environment rather than genes and that the membrane of the cell is its brain not the chromosomes.[iii] This is quite contrary to the understanding promoted by current teachings. The new understanding that you are energy and influenced by your perceptions changes how you view the possibilities of changing your biology. This new direction of thinking promotes awareness that the health of the cells has more to do with thoughts generated by your belief systems learned through environmental influence than the DNA you inherited from your parents. This knowledge returns the power to you to alter your disease course.

Our lifelong learning takes place through our belief system which generates thoughts and feelings that contribute to the function, and ultimately the healthiness, of our cells. To change your health, you must change the beliefs that impact your feelings and contribute to your thoughts. You create your world from the inside out so monitoring and taking responsibility for your thoughts will change your energy and ultimately your health. Peaceful, harmonious thoughts create a peaceful, harmonious environment on a cellular level.

Another way to encourage healthy body function from an energetic standpoint is energy efficiency. There is much focus these days on energy efficiency as it relates to the environment. The external world is a reflection of internal awareness. Internal energy efficiency can be improved by disconnecting from inherited belief systems and tuning into the power of your heart wisdom. This is the choice to disconnect from power generated by old, restrictive ancestral beliefs that are not congruent with your heart. When incongruent energy is replaced by your heartfelt wisdom, it becomes the source of power in your life. And when the power source is your heart, you flow with the natural rhythm of the Universe.

One of the undeniable results of my many years of study and experience with the heart is the awareness that the heart is intimately connected with every aspect of your total being – body, mind, emotion, and spirit. The emotional and mental aspects are just as important to address as the physical. When all these components are addressed, your spirit can soar. From my experience, the potential for healing on all levels is very real.

The power generated by your heart connection is a clear, clean energy and produces no by-products of incongruent energy. Conversely, the power generated by belief systems passed down through generations has many negative by-products — the primary one being fear. I encourage you to go beyond your thoughts and align with the wisdom of your heart; for in this newfound heart connection, you will more readily hear the whispers of your heart, and it is here you will master *The Art of Heart Healing*.

For further information about Pam and how The Art of Heart-Healing can be applied in your life, you can contact Pam at:

pamperkins@embarqmail.com or

(713) 922 0350 or visit her website at

www.theartofhearthealing.com.

Suggested Reading

The Biology of Belief by Bruce Lipton

Healing Heart by Norman Cousins

The Heartmath Solution by Doc Childre and Howard Martin

The Heart's Code: Tapping the Wisdom and Power of Our Heart Energy by Paul Pearsall

The Secret Life of Plants by Peter Tompkins and Christopher Bird

There is also an excellent article in Wikipedia called "Plant Consciousness"

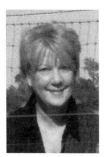

About the Author

Pamala Perkins began her nursing career and her passion to help others heal their hearts in 1967. As fate would have it that was a couple of years after coronary care units came into being in the US. She has had the benefit of seeing the full perspective of the evolution of heart care over nearly half a century.

Coronary care units were vastly different in the early years. They have gone from focusing on maintaining life while the disease process progressed to proactively intervening to prevent permanent heart damage and restore normal function when possible.

Pamala's life work as a critical care nurse was not only to give the best care she could give but to teach patients about their disease and the options available to them. She discovered if people had clear, detailed information about their conditions, they could make choices that were best for them specifically. In the medical field, this is known as informed consent.

However she found sometimes decisions are made based on limited understanding and is even sometimes influenced by someone else's agenda. The more understanding one has about the disease process, the more complete the informed consent.

The intent of *The Art of Heart Healing* is to help you understand your disease and how best to achieve healing with grace. Pamala has a private practice and sees clients on an individual basis to help them understand the underlying emotions and then facilitates the clearing of those emotions energetically. She has an office in Kingwood, TX and also does long distance healing sessions by phone. Additionally, she is available to teach these concepts to interested groups.

Her website is: www.theartofhearthealing.com and

contact info is: pamperkins@embarqmail.com

or 1- (713) 922 0350

References

[i] Science Of The Heart, HeartMath Research Center, 2001 Institute of HeartMath

[ii] The New England Journal of Medicine, Feb10, 2005

[iii] YouTube, Bruce Lipton's Latest Training,123 longevity, updated April 24,2011

16288838R00048

Made in the USA
Charleston, SC
13 December 2012